I love my Toothbrush!
Pocket Dental Coloring Book

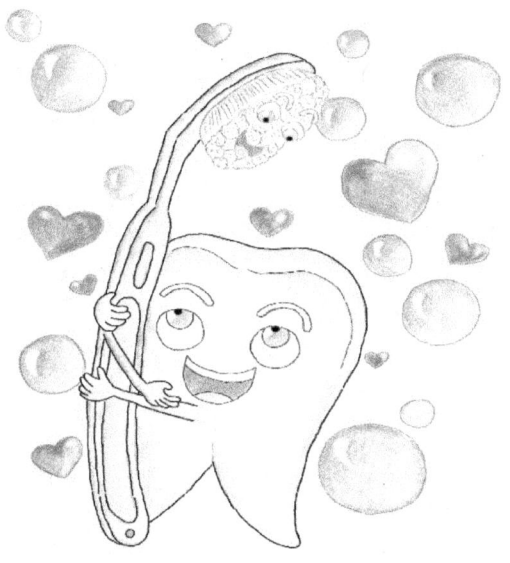

Alena Knezevic DMD, MS, PhD

Illustrated By Rina Risnawati

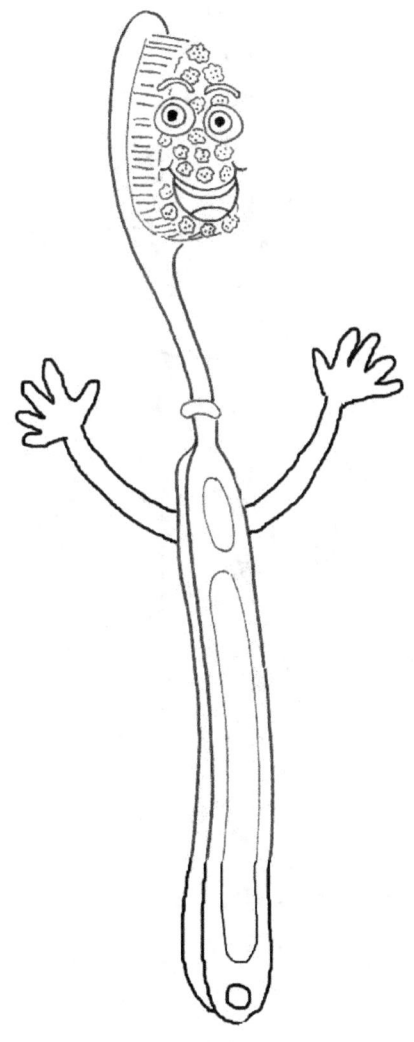

Hi there! Let me introduce myself. My name is brush – Toothbrush!

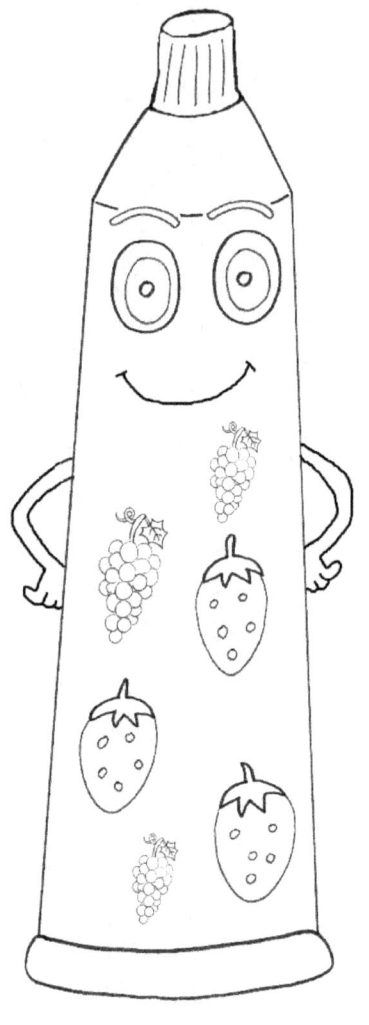

Hello ... and my name is paste - Toothpaste!

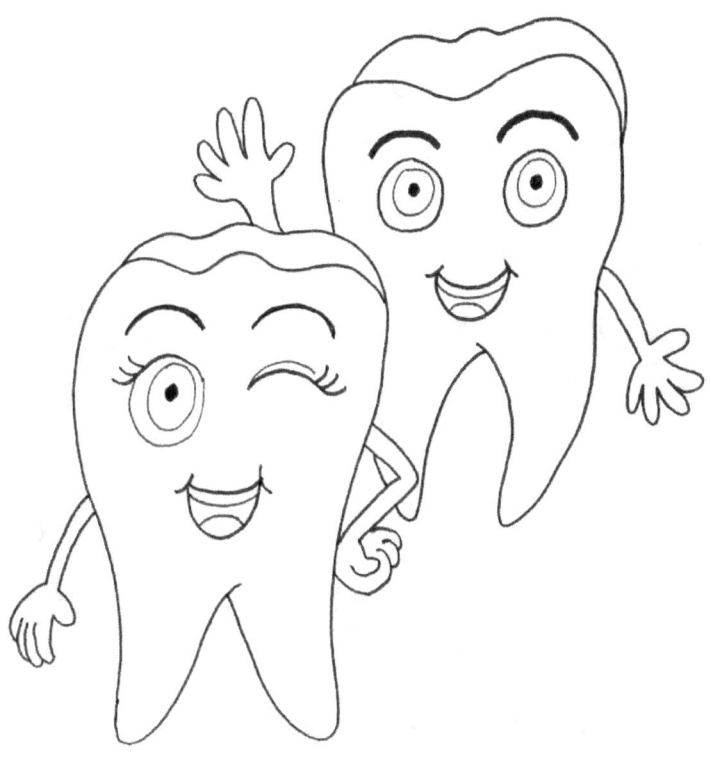

Well, well, well ... and do you know who we are?
We are your teeth – the teeth that help you to chew food, make sounds while you are speaking and make your smile beautiful!

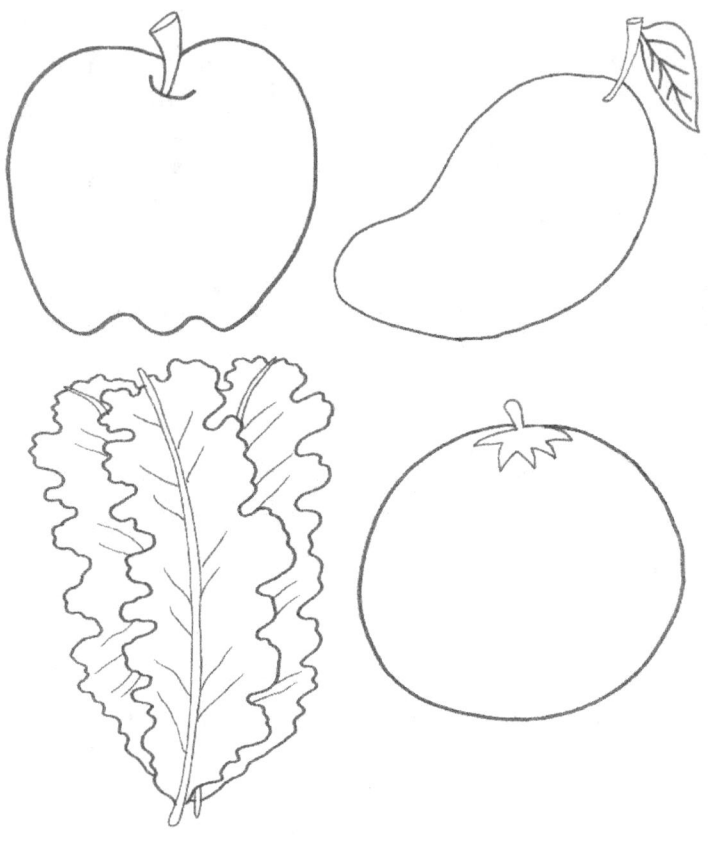

You have to keep us clean and feed yourself
and us with healthy food. Eat a lot of fruits and
vegetables!

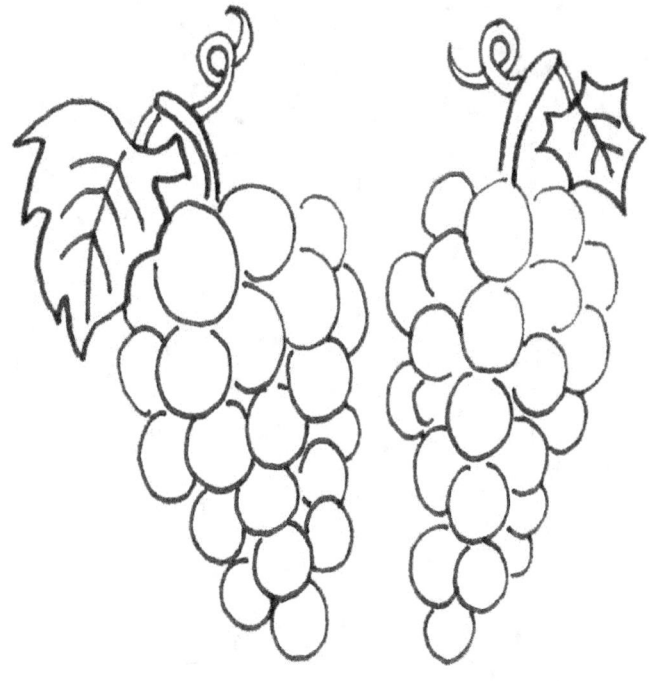

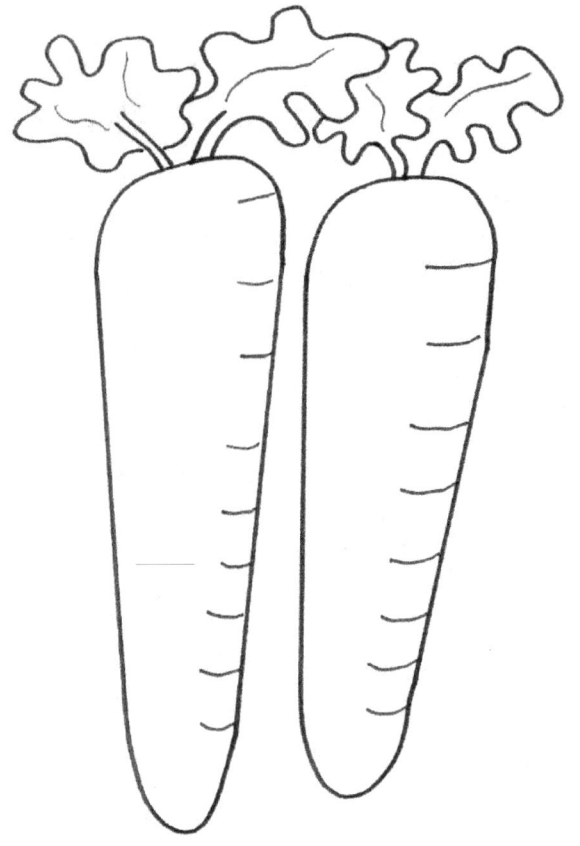

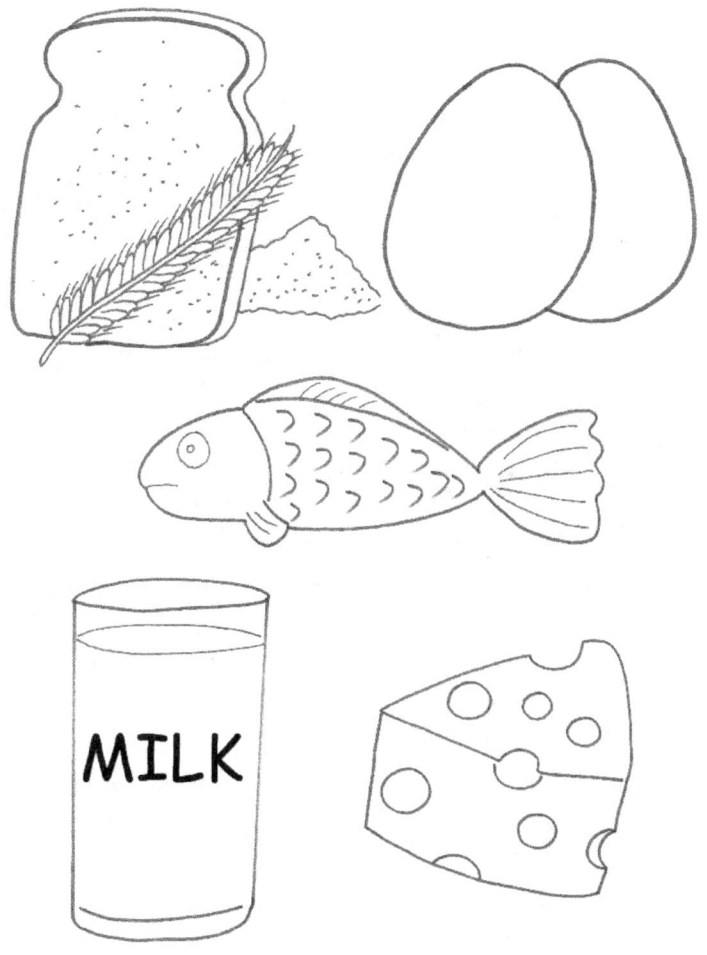

Eat a lot of proteins and whole grain foods!

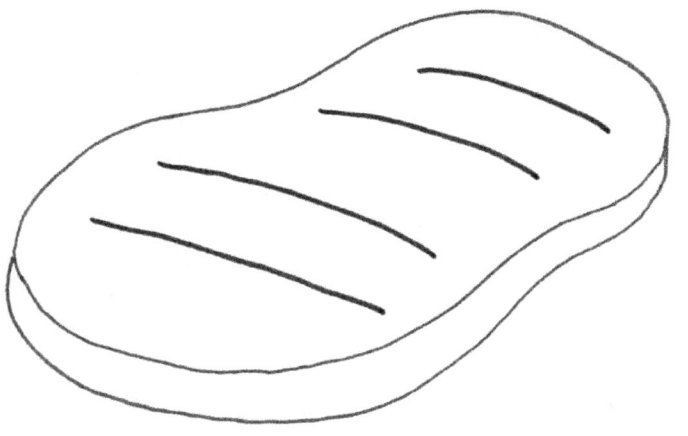

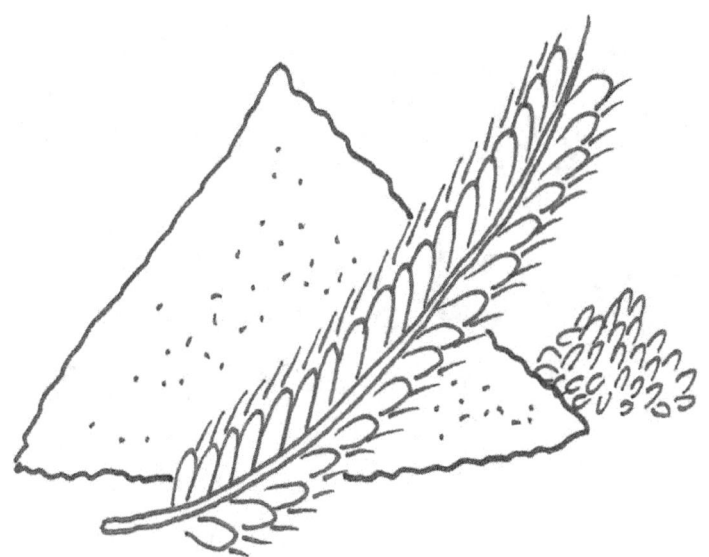

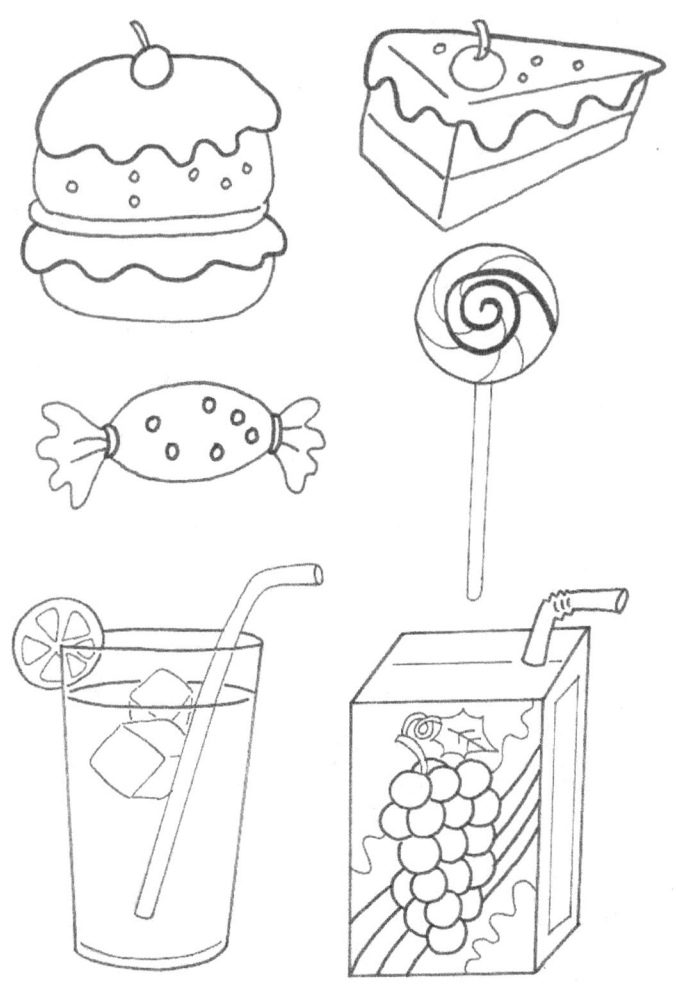

But avoid eating too many cookies and candies ... and sugared drinks as well!

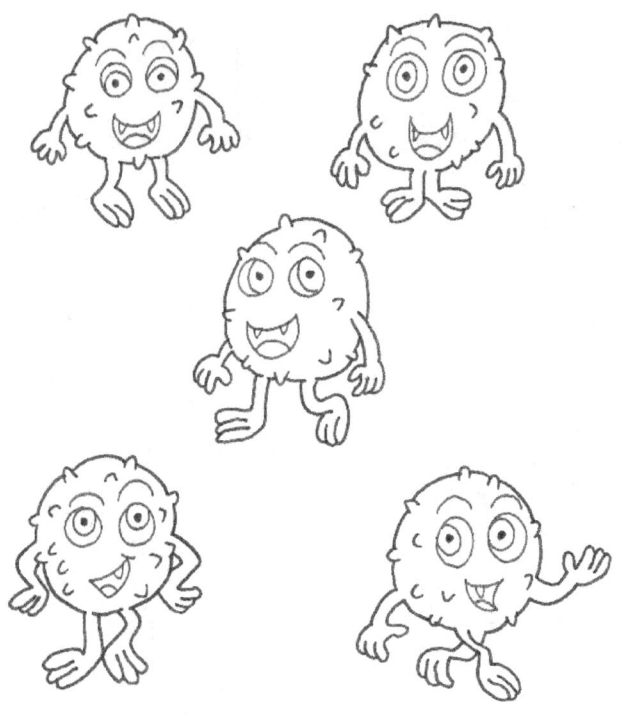

Hi there, we forgot to introduce ourselves!

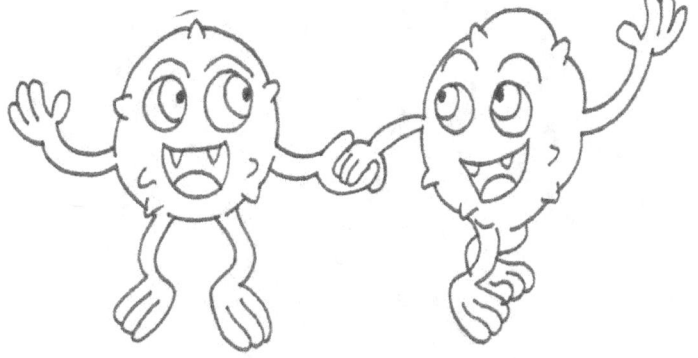

Do you know who we are?

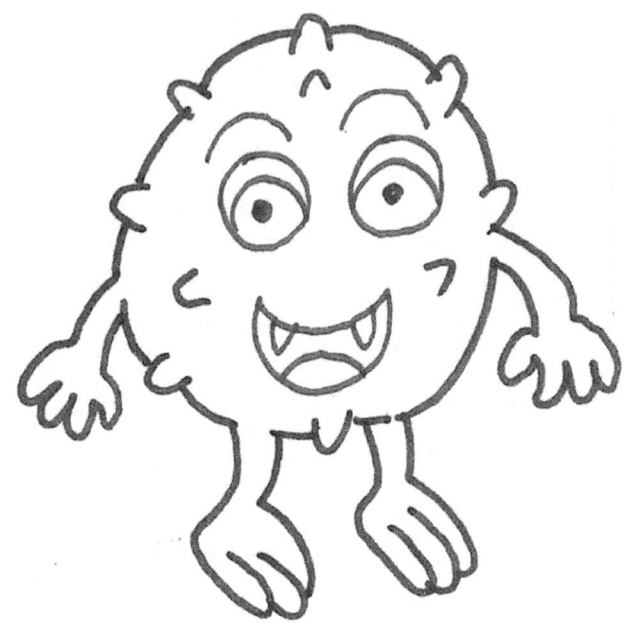

We are bacteria and we start to get very, very active and very, very happy if you do not brush your teeth and if you eat a lot of sweets.

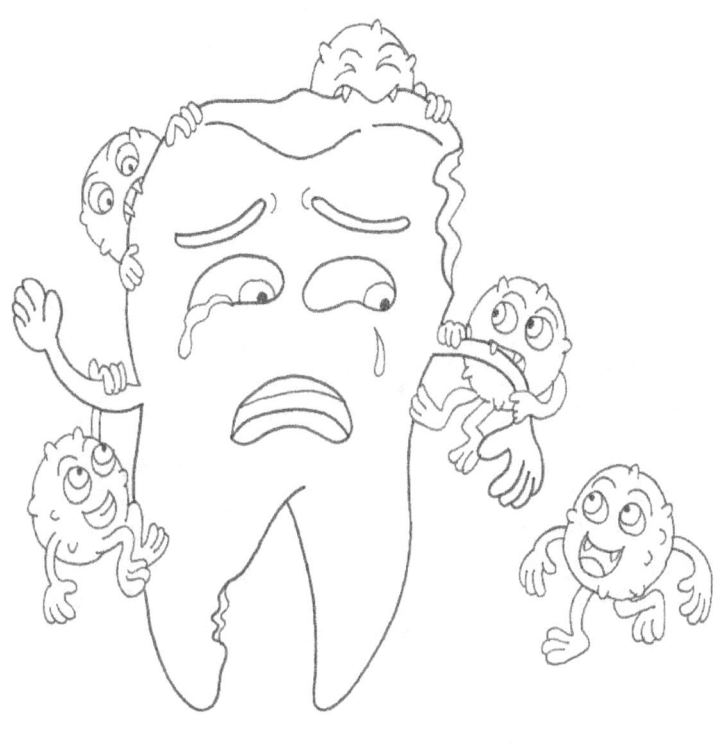

If you do not clean your teeth we will eat all the food and sweets left on your teeth ... and your teeth as well! What a party!!!

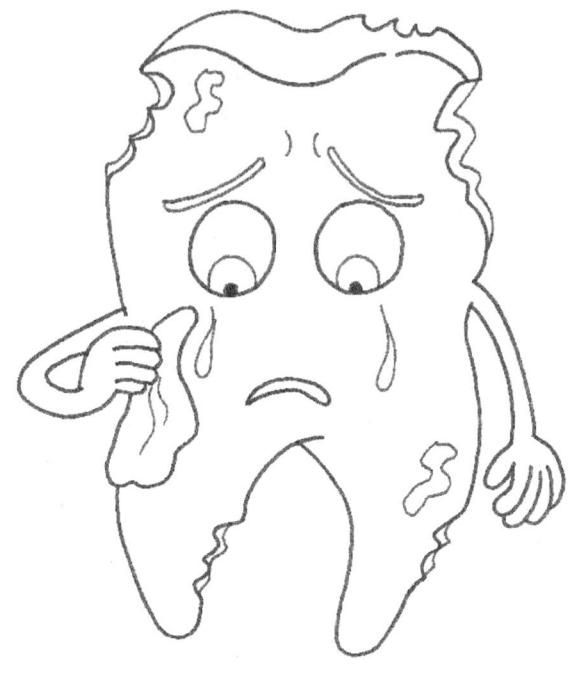

The food residue around your teeth together with bacteria will make your tooth sick if you do not brush your teeth properly. When the tooth is sick that means that you have tooth caries or tooth decay.

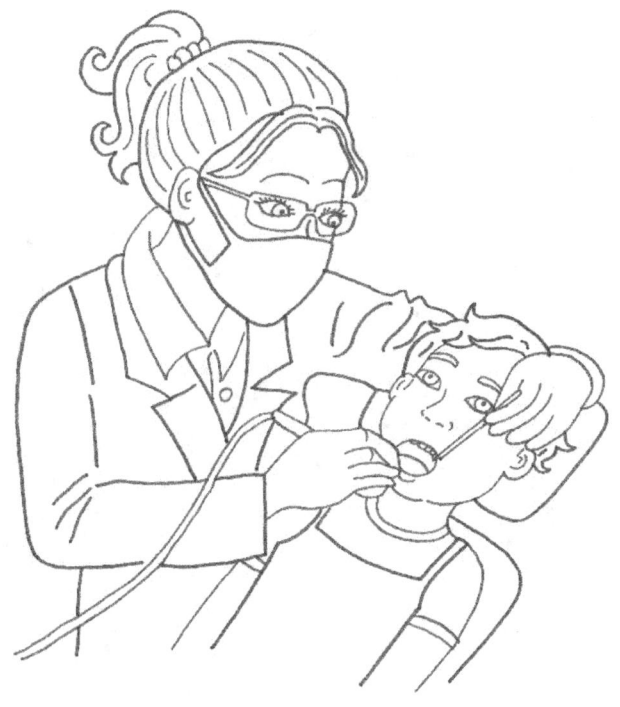

When that happens you have to visit your dentist.

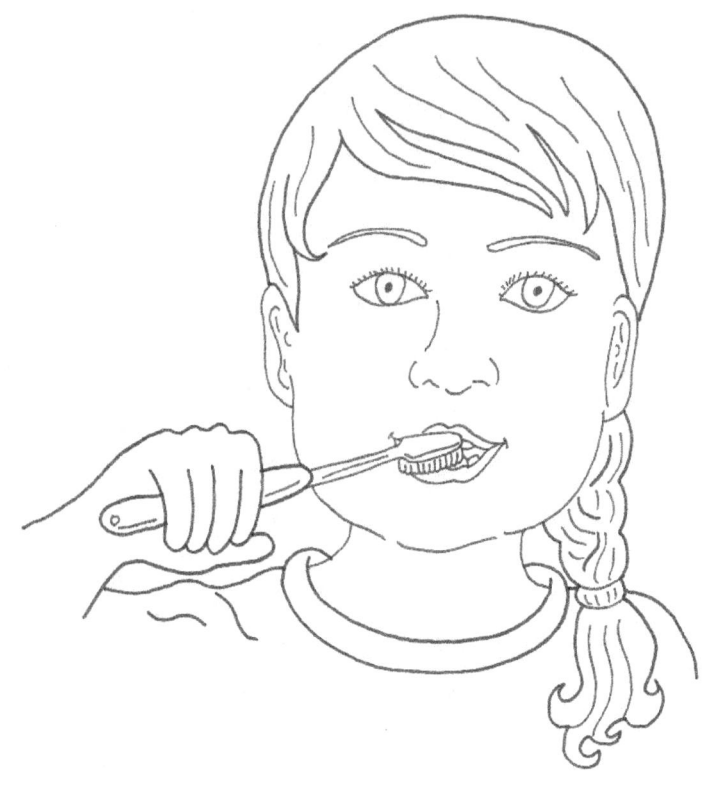

In order to make your teeth healthy you have
to brush them at least twice a day.

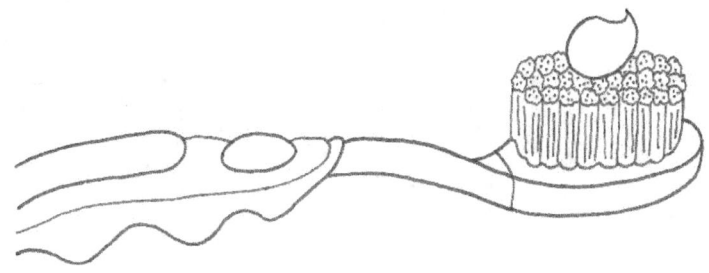

Put a pea size of paste or even less on the dry
toothbrush and brush each tooth carefully.

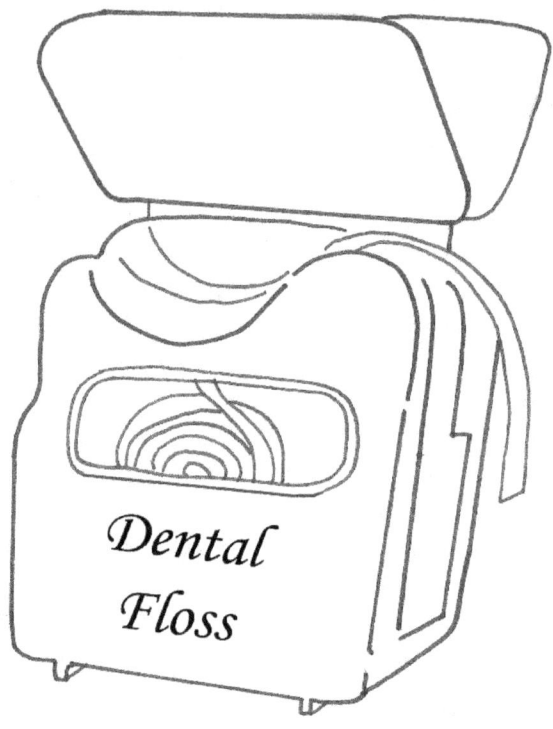

Do not forget to floss between each tooth!

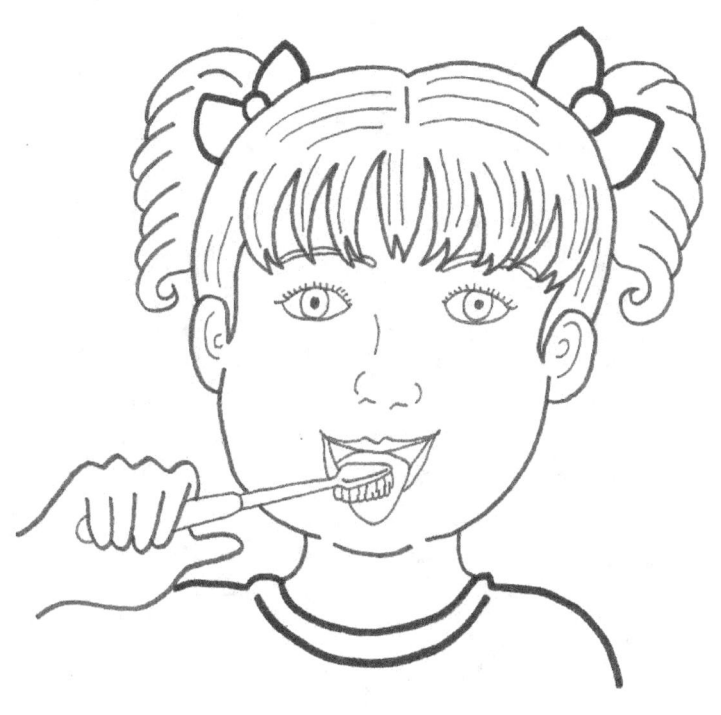

And do not forget to clean your tongue as
well! Your tongue has to be clean the same
way your teeth are.

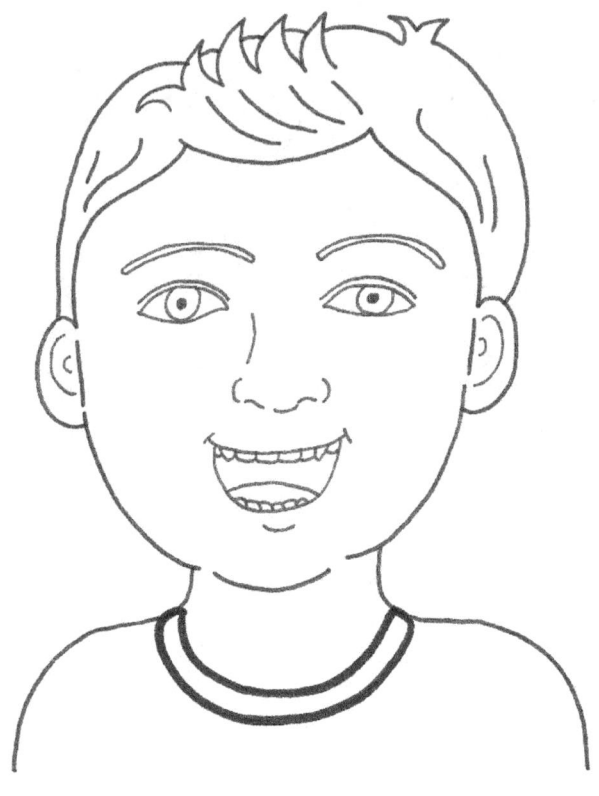

Just continue to keep your teeth clean and show to everyone your happy and beautiful smile!

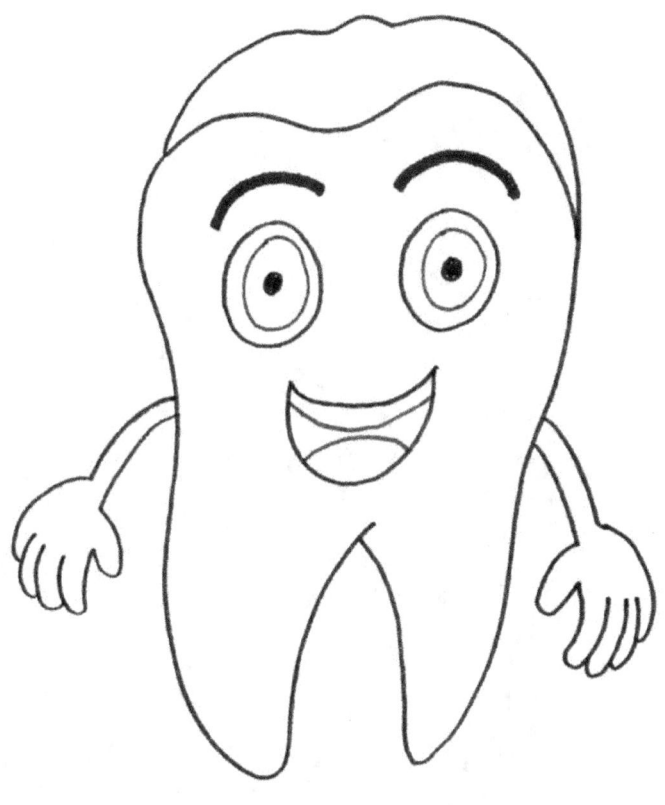

You will be happy and your teeth will be happy as well!

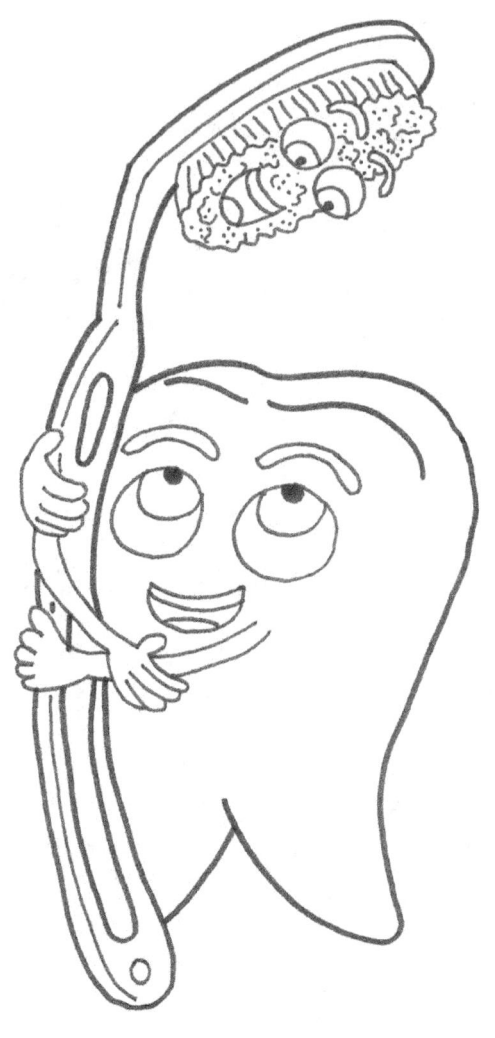

I love you!!!

Your notes ...